THE HANDBOOK
for
Credentialing Healthcare Providers

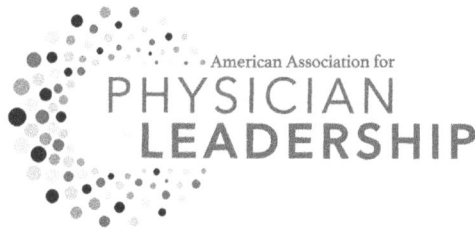

American Association for
PHYSICIAN LEADERSHIP

Ellis M. "Mac" Knight, MD, MBA, FACP, FACHE, FHM
COKER GROUP

Published by **American Association for Physician Leadership, Inc.**
PO Box 96503 | BMB 97493 | Washington, DC 20090-6503

Website: www.physicianleaders.org

AAPL books are available at special quantity discounts to use as premiums and sales promotions, or for use in corporate training programs. For more information, please write to Special Sales at journal@physicianleaders.org

This publication is designed to provide general information and is sold with the understanding that neither the author nor the publisher is engaged in rendering legal, accounting, ethical, or clinical advice. If legal or other expert advice is required, the services of a competent professional person should be sought.

13   8 7 6 5 4 3 2 1

Copyedited, typeset, indexed, and printed in the United States of America

PUBLISHER
Nancy Collins

EDITORIAL ASSISTANT
Jennifer Weiss

DESIGN & LAYOUT
Carter Publishing Studio

COPYEDITOR
Shannon Lee

Table of Contents

ABOUT THE AUTHOR

Ellis M. "Mac" Knight, MD, MBA, FACP, FACHE, FHM

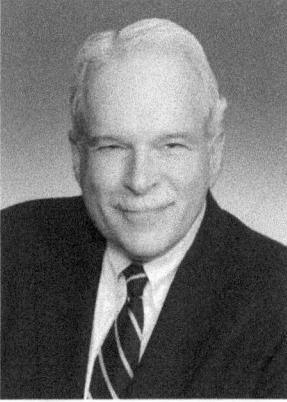

Mac Knight is senior vice president and chief medical officer of Coker Group. With over 30 years in the healthcare arena, he has attained significant experience and knowledge in this industry.

Before joining Coker, Dr. Knight served as the chief physician and clinical integration officer for Palmetto Health in Columbia, South Carolina, where he oversaw Palmetto Health's employed physician network and helped to develop and manage their clinical integration program, the Palmetto Health Quality Collaborative. Previously, he served as Palmetto Health Richland's vice president for medical affairs.

Dr. Knight graduated from Stanford University with a BA degree in human biology and received his degree, cum laude, in medicine from the University of Oregon Health Science Center's School of Medicine. He earned an MBA from the University of Massachusetts at Amherst and holds fellowships in the American College of Physicians, the Society of Hospital Medicine, and the American College of Healthcare Executives. Currently, he has an appointment as an assistant clinical professor of medicine at the University of South Carolina's School of Medicine in Columbia.

Dr. Knight oversees Coker Group's hospital strategy and operations services, and he serves as Coker Group's chief medical officer. He has a particular interest and expertise in population health management, clinical care process design, cost accounting, and hospital-physician integration.

ABOUT THE CONTRIBUTORS

JEFFRY GORKE, MBA

Jeff brings over 26 years of healthcare experience to the position of senior vice president with Coker Group. His primary focus is strategic and operational work assisting clients in macro- and micro-structural change to enhance processes and programs, drive efficiencies, and improve profitability. Jeff uses his experience to help clients with operational assessments of hospitals' and physicians' practices, physician compensation reviews, employed physician network turnarounds, financial and revenue cycle assessments, and strategic planning.

During his career, Jeff has provided management assistance and advisement to both large and small health systems, academic medical centers, and privately held physician medical groups; and he was a member of a practice management advisory board for a large pharmaceutical company. He has a successful record of designing, operationalizing, and implementing strategic initiatives to improve overall performance for clients, helping them prepare for impending shifts in care delivery and reimbursement models. Specifically, Jeff manages strategic and operational components concurrently to improve planning, governance, and top-line management while assuring operational sustainability by driving programs from efficient day-to-day management to billing and collections and data mining for physician groups and healthcare systems. Jeff has also led in the selection and implementation of electronic medical records systems (EMRs) and used data mining for clinical efficiency and financial modeling. Jeff quantifies his engagements by empowering clients to measure their outcomes and gauge their returns on investment while managing their projects.

Jeff attained a BBA from Temple University in Philadelphia and an MBA from the University of Richmond in Virginia. He is a member of the Healthcare Financial Management Association, the Medical Group Management Association, and the American College of Healthcare Executives.

ELIZABETH HARRELL

A certified medical administrative assistant, Elizabeth began her career as a billing and coding specialist in a single specialty, large-group practice. She joined Coker Group seven years ago, and her job responsibilities entail providing initial and ongoing credentialing services for Coker clients. Her work is high volume, averaging 130 providers a year.

Working with insurers in a fast-paced industry, Elizabeth is always surprised about the insurance companies' expectations and ever-changing requirements for the providers' applications. To handle the volume of her assignments and to complete her tasks accurately and on time, she has developed comprehensive tools for gathering data as well as thorough tracking instruments to stay abreast of providers' statuses.

BRENDA MATTHEWS

In her 25 years working in healthcare, Brenda Mathews has amassed expertise in all areas of practice management, including personnel management, finance and operations, and marketing and development. Specifically, she specializes in development and application of personnel policies and procedures, performance evaluation and salary review of management personnel, budget preparation, financial monitoring, operational audits, practice start-ups and expansions, marketing initiatives, and selection and implementation of capital equipment.

Her experience encompasses serving as senior administrator for a 32-provider cardiology practice, director of field operations for a practice management company, vice president of practice management services for Anesthesia, and interim central billing office director for a 40-physician multiple-specialty group. Also, she has been interim practice administrator for a free-standing cancer center, as well as director of a free-standing surgical center. Other assignments include oversight of multiple new practice start-ups, integration of 23 providers with a large hospital system, development and analysis of fee schedules, assessing and improving staffing and organization, oversight of new facility construction and renovation, and revenue analyses.

Brenda is a senior associate for Coker Group and a member of the Medical Group Management Association and the Cardiology Leaders Alliance. She studied at Florida State University in Tallahassee.

ANNETTE SULLIVAN, RHIA, AHIMA APPROVED ICD-10 CM/PCS TRAINER

As a senior manager with Coker Group, Annette is primarily involved with developing Coker's clinical documentation improvement services. Also, she participates in community needs assessments, revenue cycle reviews, medical staff strategic planning, coding audits, credentialing, information governance, electronic health records (EHRs), and other health information management system endeavors.

Annette has worked with a broad range of healthcare organizations and has experience in leading health information management functions and system clinical documentation improvement initiatives to ensure compliance and an optimal revenue stream. She has developed system-wide coding quality and correct coding initiatives and guided coding functions to maintain the integrity of the revenue cycle for a large health system in South Carolina. Also, she has directed activities related to credentialing and privileging of the medical staff and allied health personnel. She is an AHIMA Approved ICD-10 CM/PCS Trainer and has significant inpatient coding experience both at the front-line operational level and at the management and supervisory level. She is very familiar with Cerner, Meditech, PACS, Heart Lab, Dragon, and other technology used in a large health information management department.

Annette holds a BS in health information administration from the Medical University of South Carolina, Charleston, and has 28 years of health information administration experience. She has worked with several nonprofit healthcare corporations specializing in rural and urban hospital management. She is a member of the American Health Information Management Association (AHIMA).

ACKNOWLEDGMENTS

Thanks to all who have contributed their time, effort, knowledge, and experience to the writing of this book, and most of all thanks to the readers who are an often unheralded but nevertheless vital component of the American healthcare system.

We also thank our publisher and her staff, Nancy Collins and Greenbranch Publishing. We are honored for the confidence that Greenbranch continually exhibits through the many projects we have done together. Greenbranch provides the ideal opportunity for Coker Group to share our knowledge and address the concerns of healthcare entities across the nation and internationally.

Finally, the authors of this book would like to thank the countless numbers of credentialing professionals who serve to make this system work and work very successfully. Their tasks are often complex, tedious, and at times very stressful. They are nevertheless equally significant and valuable. Our hope is that this book will help make the tasks easier for those who pursue work in this field. Our objective is for the information to serve to make the system work more efficiently for all stakeholders.

Overview

Why is credentialing and privileging a medical staff important?

Credentialing ensures that clinical practitioners are duly qualified, licensed, and board certified. It reports the history of malpractice claims, state-instituted sanctions, or other undesirable professional circumstances of providers.

Credentialing and privileging of healthcare professionals protects patients and hospitals by minimizing the risk of medical errors that may result from the work of incompetent providers. It also undergirds the reputation and credibility of the institution in the eyes of providers and across the healthcare community.

Further, credentialing with insurers forms the basis for reimbursement for professional services. Without the acceptance of the professional credentials of a provider, insurers and other third-party payers will not compensate his or her claims.

Privileging ensures that clinicians are accurately credentialed and are competent to practice within a specified scope. The review is ongoing; each provider should be reviewed every two years and be issued specific privileges in writing.

The purpose of this book is to explain the necessity and to provide the process for the official documentation of each practitioner. Every chapter builds on the foundation presented in chapter 1.

- Chapter 1 introduces the credentialing topic with the quantification of its significance on the financial performance of hospitals and physician practices. The difference between medical staff credentialing of physicians and payer credentialing is explained.
- Chapter 2 outlines the how-to of medical staff credentialing and payer credentialing.
- Chapter 3 examines the pros and cons of outsourcing credentialing services.
- Chapter 4 addresses the regulations pertaining to credentialing activities and explains how they play out through peer-to-peer review.
- Chapter 5 discusses automated payer and medical staff credentialing systems, presenting guidelines for selecting products.
- Chapter 6 presents a training curriculum for those involved with credentialing activities.
- Chapter 7 wraps up the chapters with conclusions and recommendations.

The information presented in these chapters will serve as a practical resource for strengthening your organization's credentialing function.

CHAPTER 1

Credentialing—
The Foundation for Quality
and Safety

Medical credentialing, which once was straightforward and routine, has become a very important and complex task in the healthcare industry. No longer can providers simply present their academic credentials and expect to go to work and to receive reimbursement for services in a short period. Rather, their qualifications must be validated at many levels, in several areas, and at regular junctures during their careers.

Indeed, most provider and payer organizations have large teams of credentialing professionals whose full-time job it is to evaluate fully an individual's educational, training, and work history to ensure that he or she can meet the standards required to be granted practice privileges and to be paid for rendering high-quality and safe medical care.

Credentialing is an important process in two main venues: hospitals or other provider organizations, where medical staff credentialing occurs, and the healthcare marketplace, where third-party payers determine whether practitioners hold the proper credentials to be paid for delivering medical services. Although medical staff and payer credentialing involve very similar processes, they also differ somewhat, especially relative to the granting of privileges to perform certain activities. These privileges primarily fall under the purview of an organization's medical staff.

While interrelated, credentialing and licensing are separate processes that serve different purposes and are performed by separate private and public organizations.

PRACTITIONERS

Credentialing usually involves licensed medical practitioners, which can include physicians (i.e., Medical Doctors, Doctors of Osteopathy, or others with a variety of degrees who have been licensed by the state to practice medicine), dentists, clinical psychologists, podiatrists, and other provider types as determined by the organization responsible for the credentialing process.

Recent years have shown growth in numbers in the licensing and credentialing of advanced practice nurses (i.e., nurse practitioners) and physician assistants. For credentialers, this increase has become a major undertaking because these types of providers

1

work, in most states, under the direct supervision of a licensed physician. Instead of the responsibility to maintain the credentials of one professional, the work increases exponentially with the additional licensed professionals.

RISK AND LIABILITY

Underlying the credentialing process is the desire to protect the public from those who do not have adequate education, training, and experience or the demonstrated competency to deliver high-quality, safe healthcare services. Unfortunately, several widely publicized cases have been reported of extremely dangerous, even homicidal, physicians who were able to succeed repetitively in passing through the credentialing process until caught. Perhaps even more disturbing than these high-profile cases, however, are the many practitioners who are now credentialed to practice medicine but are doing so unsafely or with poor quality standards.

A thorough and systematic approach to the credentialing process that uses industry-wide best practices and standards should help prevent or mitigate the validation problem. Also, providers themselves, especially physicians, need to take their obligation seriously both to hold themselves to the highest standards and to hold their peers to the same standards. Physicians and other providers must work tirelessly to assure that those who are incompetent are removed from the system. This task is not easy, nor should the responsibility for policing provider competencies strictly rest with organizations, such as the organized medical staff's credentialing committee. Nevertheless, no group is better equipped to assess another's capabilities than the professional peers of the provider type in question. Practitioners need to take the responsibility very seriously to hold their fellow professionals accountable and set standards for the industry that ensure that the utmost priorities are high-quality care and patient safety.

The governing board of most hospitals and healthcare systems has the ultimate responsibility of ensuring that medical staff credentialing is done appropriately. The responsibility for verification standards cannot be simply delegated to the medical staff. Increasingly, lay board members realize that they must become familiar with credentialing regulations, standards, policies, and procedures. While most board members are financially protected through directors' and officers' insurance from personal liability for inadequate credentialing activities, this protection does not extend to regulatory sanctions that might be brought against an organization whose board members are not adequately overseeing the credentialing process.

AUTOMATION OF CREDENTIALING PROCESSES

Credentialing is a time-consuming, laborious task that is often perceived by key stakeholders to take far too long to perform. Automated tools, therefore, are available to speed this process along and to accelerate some of the credentialing steps. However, that automation is only appropriate for certain noncritical credentialing tasks, and human resources must still make sure that items such as primary source verification are done thoroughly and appropriately.

POLICIES AND PROCEDURES

What follows in this book are multiple details regarding best practices in the credentialing process. These best practices should be codified in the individual organizations and followed consistently. Variability from written procedures undermines high-quality credentialing activities and can lead to serious harm events in the patient care arena. Furthermore, and as mentioned, many credentialing processes require seemingly unacceptable lengths of time to properly perform. Nevertheless, certain steps in the process should not be subjected to shortcuts. Most high-performing credentialing offices are adequately staffed and equipped to handle the workload in a high-quality fashion that does not overly prolong the process.

GOING FORWARD

Finally, credentialing is a dynamic process, and while this book attempts to give the reader the most up-to-date information possible, new requirements and further development of best practices will require all credentialing professionals continuously to update and expand their knowledge. That said, the contributors to this book hope to give the reader a solid grounding in the basics of medical staff credentialing that proves to be of value to those involved in this highly important work.

CHAPTER 2

Types of Credentialing

Effective medical staff credentialing and privileging is a critical component of a health-care provider's success in providing safe and effective patient care. It is extremely important to have a succinct and systematic process that ensures that all licensed inde-pendent practitioners granted the privilege of taking care of patients are competent to do so with the education, professionalism, and experience necessary to provide quality outcomes. If an organization fails to perform due diligence in acquiring and maintaining proficient medical staff members, it can be detrimental to patient satisfaction, revenue, and risk management.

Healthcare organizations that have standardized and streamlined credentialing and privileging policies and procedures fare better than organizations that deviate from policy, depending on extenuating circumstances. It is imperative to establish con-sistent policies and procedures to manage the credentialing process and to abide by them. The policies and procedures should include, but are not limited to, medical staff rules and bylaws, credentialing policies and procedures, and privileging criteria. These guiding principles will ensure that the organized medical staff is equipped with all of the necessary mechanisms to appoint, manage, and maintain medical staff member-ship and clinical privileges. The oversight of the credentialing policies and procedures must rest with the credentialing committee, the medical executive committee, and the governing board.

MEDICAL STAFF CREDENTIALING

A complete screening and review process must be carried out each and every time for the initial appointment and for reappointment of medical staff to ensure that only quali-fied, competent practitioners provide patient care. This information should begin with a formal application that includes the following:

- applicant's training;
- background;
- references;
- clinical experience;
- certification;
- licensure status;
- professional liability insurance and claims history; and
- evidence of current competence or requested privileges and performance data.

Primary source verification must be conducted to ensure that all information provided by the practitioner is accurate. All gaps in practice and employment must be scrutinized and validated to prevent providing privileges to high-risk and negligent providers. The organized medical staff may delegate the administrative and daily management functions of credentialing to highly trained credentialing staff but must remain engaged throughout the process and recognize that the responsibility rests with them and the entities outlined above. Active participation in peer-to-peer references may be necessary at times to ensure that only qualified practitioners gain access to the medical staff. The medical staff must evaluate evidence of unusual patterns or excess numbers of professional liability actions, resulting in a final judgment.

It is also good form to verify that all applicants are not excluded from the Medicare, Medicaid, or other federal healthcare programs.

Instituting rigorous policies that limit or prevent expediting medical staff privileges will mitigate risks and alleviate unnecessary pressures placed on individuals charged with providing privileges to the medical staff. Temporary privileging for staff and locum tenems should have strict parameters that delineate who are eligible along with the circumstances when such privileges are warranted. The credentialing process should never be shortened to accommodate requests for temporary privileges. Effective, streamlined credentialing procedures coupled with adequate planning and coordination with medical staff recruiters, department chiefs ,and the leadership team should all but negate the need for temporary privileges except for urgent patient care needs or a shortage of critical resources.

The Joint Commission Accreditation Standards

Credentialing procedures, as mandated by The Joint Commission (TJC), require at a minimum the following:

- Information specific to the applicant's current licensure status, training, and current competence must be collected by the hospital using a defined credentialed process that is based on medical staff recommendations, approved by the governing body, and documented in the medical staff bylaws. Verification must be in writing and must come from the primary source, if possible, or from a credentials verification organization (CVO). The identity of the applicant must be verified. This verfication can be accomplished by viewing either a current hospital picture identification card (ID) or a valid picture ID issued by a state or a federal agency such as a driver's license or passport.
- The medical staff must review and analyze all relevant information received regarding current licensure status, training, experience, current competence, and ability to perform the requested privileges through a clearly defined process. The organization develops and consistently applies criteria that will be considered in the decision to grant, limit, or deny a requested privilege. These criteria are based on recommendations from the medical staff and are approved by the governing body. Criteria must directly relate to the quality of healthcare, treatment, and services that have been evaluated. The governing body or its delegated committee has final authority for granting, renewing, or denying privileges. Privileges cannot exceed two years.

- The privileging decision must be communicated to the requesting practitioner within a timeframe specified in the medical staff bylaws. In the case of a denial, the applicant must be told the reason for denial. The privileging decision must be distributed and made available to all appropriate internal and/or external persons or entities, as defined by the organization and applicable law. The practitioner must be notified of available due process or, when applicable, the option to implement the fair hearing and appeal process. If it chooses, the governing body can use an expedited process for making initial appointments and reappointments to the medical staff and for granting privileges. The governing body may delegate these decisions to a committee consisting of at least two voting governing body members. Expedited credentialing may not be used if the applicant's application is incomplete, or if the medical staff executive committee makes a final recommendation that is adverse or has limitations. Criteria developed by the medical staff for the expedited process must be followed.
- The following situations should be evaluated on an individual basis and would usually lead to ineligibility for expedited credentialing. It should be noted that these issues do not immediately render a practitioner ineligible because TJC allows the organization to consider each specific case.
  - The applicant has a current or previously successful challenge to licensure or registration.
  - The applicant has had an involuntary termination of medical staff membership or involuntary limitation, reduction, denial, or loss of clinical privileges.
  - The applicant has had an unusual pattern of, or an excessive number of, professional liability actions that resulted in a final judgment.
- The medical staff must have a fair hearing and appeal process for addressing adverse decisions regarding reappointment, denial, reduction, suspension, or revocation of privileges that relate to quality of care, treatment, and service issues. A fair hearing and appeals process allows the practitioner the opportunity to defend himself or herself against the adverse action before an unbiased hearing panel of the medical staff. Also, the practitioner can appeal the decision of the hearing panel to the governing body. The hearing and appeals procedure must be fair and must include a mechanism to schedule a hearing, procedures for the hearing to follow, the composition of the hearing committee as a committee of impartial peers, and a governing body mechanism to appeal adverse decisions. The process may differ for medical staff members and those nonmembers who are granted privileges.
- The medical staff makes recommendations to the governing body for medical staff appointment as part of its oversight of the quality of care, treatment, and services provided by privileged practitioners. The medical staff must develop and use criteria for medical staff membership. These criteria should be designed to assure the medical staff and governing body that patients will receive quality care, treatment, and services. Appointments and subsequent reappointments cannot exceed a period of two years.
- The medical staff must obtain and evaluate peer recommendations when considering appointment and initial granting of privileges and when considering termi-

nation from the medical staff, revision, or revocation of clinical privileges. Peer recommendations are obtained from a practitioner in the same professional discipline as the applicant with personal knowledge of the applicant's ability to practice. A physician must provide the peer recommendation for a physician, a dentist for a dentist, and so on. According to TJC, appropriate sources for peer recommendations include the following:

— an organization's performance-improvement committee, the majority of whose members are the applicant's peers;

— reference letter(s), written documentation, or documented telephone conversation(s) about the applicant from a peer(s) who is knowledgeable about the applicant's professional performance and competence;

— a department or clinical service chairperson who is a peer; or

— the medical staff executive committee.

- On renewal of privileges, if there are insufficient practitioner-specific data available, the medical staff can use and evaluate peer recommendations. Peer recommendations must address relevant training, experience, current competence, and any effects of health status on privileges being requested. Also, peer recommendations must include evaluation of the applicant's medical knowledge, technical and clinical skills, clinical judgment, communication skills, interpersonal skills, and professionalism.

- Issuing temporary clinical privileges can fulfill an important patient care need. For example, if the only physician privileged to perform a highly specialized service becomes ill, disabled, or is otherwise unable to perform this service, a qualified physician may be brought in and given temporary privileges to provide this service while his or her credentials are being reviewed for medical staff membership and delineated clinical privileges. In another example, a recently recruited applicant whose specialized training is needed to perform necessary procedures may be given temporary privileges while his or her credentials are being processed.

- TJC standards allow the chief executive officer (CEO) or his or her authorized designee to grant temporary privileges based on the recommendation of the president of the medical staff or authorized designee.

- TJC recognizes two circumstances for which the granting of temporary privileges to a licensed independent practitioner would be acceptable: 1) to fulfill an important patient care, treatment, and service need, or 2) when an applicant with a complete, clean application that raises no concerns is awaiting review and approval of the medical staff executive committee and the governing body.

— There are specific requirements for each circumstance.

— Temporary privileges may be granted when there is an important patient care need that mandates an immediate authorization to practice. These privileges are granted for a limited period as determined by the bylaws.

— In these circumstances, temporary privileges may be granted by the CEO upon the recommendation of the president of the medical staff. Current licensure and current competence must be verified before the granting of privileges. The Healthcare Quality Improvement Act (HQIA) requires the healthcare entity to query the National Practitioner Data Bank (NPDB) before granting privileges; and individual states and hospitals may have additional requirements. The medical staff bylaws must document a time period that these privileges would be in effect, and this time limit must be followed.

— For the new applicant, privileges may be granted by the CEO upon the recommendation of the president of the medical staff. Temporary privileges may only be granted for up to 120 days. Before granting privileges, there must be verification of current licensure, relevant training or experience, current competence, and any other criteria required by the organization's medical staff bylaws. The NPDB query results must have been obtained and evaluated. It is also required that the new applicant has a complete application with no current or previously successful challenge to licensure or registration, has not been subject to involuntary termination of medical staff appointment at another organization, and has not been subject to involuntary limitation, reduction, denial, or loss of clinical privileges.

- All licensed independent practitioners and other practitioners privileged through the medical staff process must participate in continuing education. An individual's participation in continuing education must be documented and considered at reappointment and at renewal or revision of privileges. Hospital-sponsored educational activities must be prioritized by the medical staff. These activities should relate, at least in part, to the type and nature of care, treatment, and services offered by the hospital and to the findings of performance-improvement activities.

Summary of Medical Staff Credentialing

It is essential to empower those involved with credentialing with completely standardized information that is uniformly presented in a timeframe that allows enough time to consider carefully all of the necessary aspects of medical staff membership. In addition, it is necessary to design an application or reappointment packet that encompasses all of the requirements of credentialing and privileging while providing enough information to assess appropriately the qualifications and competencies of the applicant. Establishing consistent credentialing practices will provide safe patient care provided by practitioners that are qualified to achieve the best outcomes.

PAYER CREDENTIALING

Provider credentialing and enrollment is an essential step in practice management and to a provider's success. Unless the right steps are taken to credential a provider, the provider will not be able to bill the insurance company. Credentialing involves the process of obtaining a provider's information and using this information to complete the needed applications. The applications are then sent to the insurance companies and tracked for their enrollment. A provider cannot start billing until the applicants have been credentialed correctly. One of the most integral parts of the credentialing process is the collection and verification of vital data from the provider regarding his or her education, training, experience, practice history, location, disclosure of any issues impacting his or her ability to provide care, and other background information.

National Provider Identifier

Currently providers are identified by numbers called National Provider Identifiers (NPIs). If a provider does not have this number, he or she will need to apply for it at the National Plan and Provider Enumeration System (NPPES) Web site (https://nppes.cms.hhs.gov). The NPI number was created to replace an older provider tracking number called the Universal Provider Identification Number (UPIN). Some providers have an NPI and a UPIN, but most payers do not use the older tracking number. If your provider has a group, he or she may choose to create an NPI for that group, which would be Type 2, leaving the individual provider to be Type 1. After the provider has obtained an NPI number, he or she can start gathering the remaining information to enter into a provider application.

When meeting with a new provider, the credentialer should have a list of necessary items to get started in the credentialing process, including updated licenses and updated curriculum vitae (with dates and months). All payers will require an up-to-date state license; controlled substance certificate (if applicable); and U.S. Department of Justice, Drug Enforcement Agency (DEA) and liability face sheet. The credentialer must verify effective dates and expiration dates on all licenses and certifications to see if renewals are needed. A checklist of required documents is available as Figure 2.1.

FIGURE 2.1: Checklist of Required Documents

Received	Document
	Copy of State Medical License—including *renewal* receipt, pocket copy, and wall certificate
	Copy of Medical School Diploma (MD, DO, DPM) *or* Certificate (NP, PA, CRNA, etc.)
	Copy of Federal DEA certificate with *current* office address—receipt from website is okay (www.deadiversion.usdoj.gov)
	Copy of (past and present) Malpractice face sheet—including tail coverage policies
	Copy of *current* Curriculum Vitae (CV)—CV dates must show *month and year*
	Copy of current Driver's License
	Copy of provider's Controlled Substance Certificate/license, if applicable (CDS or DPS in certain states)
	Copy of Social Security Card or other official verification of SSN (clear copy)
	Copy of Board Certification or *proof* of Board Qualified/Eligible, Date expected to take exam

	Copy of Internship and Residency Certificate with dates *or* letter from Program Director
	List of *all* hospitals (with addresses) where provider has current privileges, admitting privileges status (i.e., Courtesy, Active, etc.)

Council for Affordable Quality Healthcare

The process of credentialing physicians and other healthcare providers involves considerable paperwork and administrative time, but it can be reduced by using available database resources, such as the Council for Affordable Quality Healthcare (CAQH Universal Credentialing DataSource). The CAQH is a not-for-profit collaborative alliance of the nation's leading health plans and networks. CAQH's mission is the improvement of healthcare access and quality for patients and the reduction of the administrative burden for healthcare providers and their office staff members.

The CAQH Universal Credentialing DataSource (UCD) system database is the single repository of participating health plans for healthcare provider information, alleviating the need for physicians and other healthcare providers to complete and submit many different credentialing forms for multiple health plans, hospitals, and other healthcare organizations. It is designed to simplify the credentialing process, making it easier for providers by gathering data in a single repository that may be accessed by participating health plans and other healthcare organizations. The UCD enables providers to easily update their information. CAQH works to ensure that the healthcare providers under contract health plans are adequately trained, certified, and/or licensed to provide care.

The credentialer also will need to collect providers' personal and professional information and history to complete the applications. There will be several different questions on each application that will be different from the next. If a provider already has a CAQH application set up, then you would be able to take most of your information from that application. If the provider does not have a CAQH application, you will need to have the provider fill out a provider questionnaire to get started. Below is a questionnaire comprised of questions taken from different applications to assist in gathering the necessary information.

Provider Questionnaire

- Name and Degree: _____
- Other name (Former, Maiden, etc.) _____
- Male/Female
- Home address: _____
- City, State, Zip: _____
- Contact phone number: _____
- How long have you lived at this address?: _____
- Provider e-mail: _____

- Date of Birth: _____
- Social Security Number: _____
- City, State (Country if not USA) of Birth: _____
- Primary Specialty: _____
- Effective date: _____   End date: _____
- Other Specialty: _____
- Effective date: _____   End date: _____
- Are you board certified? Y/N
- If yes, certificate #: _____
- Issue date: _____   Expiration date: _____
- If no, please list when/if you plan on taking your boards: _____
- Individual NPI: _____   Issue date: _____
- Log-in: _____   Password: _____
- License #: _____
- Effective date: _____   End date: _____
- Please list all license #s you have had and state and expiration date:

  _____

  _____

- CDS/DPS#: _____

  Effective date: _____   End date: _____
- DEA #: _____

  Effective date: _____   End date: _____
- Liability Company: _____
- Address: _____
- Phone: _____
- Policy #: _____
- Limits: _____
- Start and expiration dates: _____
- Will the office be handicapped accessible? Y/N
- What are your office hours?

Sunday	Monday	Tuesday	Wednesday	Thursday	Friday	Saturday

- Do you provide 24-hour coverage? Y/N

  If yes, please provide details: _____

  _____

- Will you have an answering service? Y/N

  Do you speak an additional language (other than English)? Y/N

  If yes, what other language(s)? _____

- ECFMG/USMILE #: _____

- UPIN (if issued): _____

- Individual Medicare #: _____ Certification date: _____

Medicare

- Name of Medical/Professional school *and* year of graduation:

  _____

  _____

- Current Practice Name: _____

- Current Practice Tax ID: _____

- Medicare # associated with current practice: _____

- Effective date and date enrolled: _____

- Current Practice Address: _____

- City, State, Zip: _____

- Date of last day with current practice: _____

- Current Hospital Affiliations and Status (active, courtesy):

  _____

  _____

  _____

- Are there any changes or additions to your current hospital affiliations?

  If yes, list the changes: _____

  _____

  _____

  _____

- Are you currently a resident or in a fellowship program? Y/N

  If yes, please provide the name and address of the facility in which you are a resident or fellow: _____

_____

_____

_____

If yes, are the services rendered at that facility regulated for graduation from that residency or fellowship program? Y/N

If yes, do you render services at other facilities or practice locations? Y/N

Date of Completion: _____

- Do you hold a doctoral degree in psychology? Y/N

  If yes, please furnish the field of your psychology degree (and attach a copy with this application).

  _____

- Individual Medicare #: _____   Certification date: _____
- Individual Medicaid #: _____
- Practice NPI: _____   Issue date: _____

  Log-in: _____   Password: _____

- If you don't have a license and are certified, please list certification #, state where issued, effective date, and expiration date: _____

  _____

  _____

Medicare Group Application

- New Practice Legal Business Name: _____

  _____

- Doing Business As: _____

  _____

- Incorporation date (if applicable): _____
- State where incorporated: _____
- New Practice Tax ID: _____
- Group/Practice Medicare #: _____
- Group/Practice Medicaid #: _____
- Does the group/practice you are joining have adverse legal history? Y/N

  If yes, please attach the information.
- Practice Address: _____
- City, State, Zip: _____

- County: _____
- Office Manager's name: _____
- New Practice Phone: _____
- Fax number: _____
- Supervising Physician's Name and NPI (if applicable): _____

  _____

- Covering Physician(s)' name, address, phone, fax, and NPI: _____

  _____

  _____

  _____

- Date you saw your first Medicare patient at this practice location:

  _____

- Is this practice location a:
  - ☐ Private practice office setting
  - ☐ Hospital
  - ☐ Retirement/assisted living community
  - ☐ Other healthcare facility: _____
- Effective date of new demographics/changes: _____
- Checks made payable to: _____
- Billing Address: _____
- City, State, Zip: _____
- Mailing Address: _____
- City, State, Zip:_____
- Special Remittance address (if any): _____

  _____

- Where would you like your remittance Notices or Special Payments sent?

  Address: _____

  _____

  _____

- Please provide the address for where your Medical records are stored.

  Address: _____

  _____

  _____

- Will you offer lab services in the office? Y/N

  If yes, please provide CLIA documentation.
- Will you file claims electronically? Y/N
- Will you be using a billing company? Y/N

  If yes, please list:

  Company Name: _____

  Phone number: _____

  Contact name: _____

  Phone number and ext.: _____

- Depository information (for electronic funds transfer)
- Name of Bank: _____
- Address: _____
- City, State, Zip: _____

  Bank contact: _____

  Name on account: _____

- Routing number: _____
- Account number: _____
- Have you ever had any adverse legal action taken against you (Malpractice Claims)? Y/N
- If yes, please attach details.
- Please list 3 professional references. (Name, address, specialty, phone, and fax)

  _____

  _____

  _____

  _____

  _____

  _____

CAQH ProView

- Are you enrolled in CAQH? Y/N

  If yes, Username: _____

  Password: _____ _ _____

  CAQH #: _____ _ _____

Medicaid

- Are you currently or have you ever been enrolled in a Medicaid Program? Y/N

- If *currently,* please check one of the following:

  ☐ Change of employment, group association, practice, or business structure.

  Change effective date: _____

  Current provider ID: _____

  ☐ Previous (former) Group

  Name: _____ _____

  Provider ID: _____

  Termination date: _____

  ☐ Additional service location

  Effective date: _____

  Current provider ID(s): _____

  ☐ Other _____

  Effective date: _____

  Provider ID: _____

- Are you enrolled in a Medicaid Vaccine for Children Program? Y/N

  If yes, VFC ID #: _____

- Please choose what you will be enrolling as:

  Individual   Group/Payee   Facility/Organization

- Please choose your Business (organization) type:

  Sole proprietor   LLC   Private

  Individual practitioner   LLP   Tribal

  Corporation   Not-for-profit   Chain

  Group   Partnership

  Estate/Trust   Public service corporation

  Government owned   Intergovernmental

  Other: _____

- If you will be using an authorized agent as your EDI submitter, please complete the following:

  Trading partner name: _____

  Trading partner phone #: _____

Federal Tax ID #: _____

NPI: _____

Taxonomy Code(s): _____

Disclosure Questions

- Have you ever had any negative action taken in connection with your license, including, but not limited to, refusal, suspension, revocation, probation reprimand, censure, or restriction in any way by any state or jurisdictional board? Y/N

- Have you ever been censured by a medical society or other professional society or other professional board or association? Y/N

- Have you ever had your Drug Enforcement Administration number (DEA #) restricted, suspended, revoked, or otherwise limited, or your DEA license application refused? Y/N

- Have you ever had an agreement with Medicare or Medicaid that was restricted, probational, suspended, excluded, or terminated? Y/N

- Have you ever been required or agreed to pay civil monetary penalties under Medicare or Medicaid? Y/N

- Have you ever been convicted of a criminal offense other than a minor traffic violation? Y/N

- Has any hospital or facility ever taken any action regarding your privileges, including, but not limited to, suspension, restriction, denial, or revocation? Y/N

- Have you ever voluntarily resigned privileges in lieu of disciplinary action? Y/N

- Has there been, within the last five years, more than one malpractice judgment found against you or malpractice settlement made, with or without prejudice, in excess of five hundred thousand ($500,000) dollars? Y/N

- Do you have an impairment, which even with reasonable accommodation would interfere with your ability to provide care according to accepted standards of professional performance, or would pose a threat to patient health and safety? Y/N

- Are you now or have you ever been an active or habitual user of any mind or mood altering substance, including, but not limited to, alcohol, narcotics, barbiturates, hypnotics, amphetamines, cocaine, benzodiazepines, or other controlled or illegal substances? Y/N

- Has your participation in any insurance carrier sponsored program been suspended or revoked? Y/N

Once you have all items to start credentialing, you can enter or update the provider's information in CAQH ProView. CAQH ProView is an online electronic application from which several private payers pull a provider's information to start the credentialing process. Medicare and Medicaid do not use CAQH ProView. You can find CAQH ProView at https://proview.caqh.org.

After you have entered the provider's information into CAQH ProView, you will need to start calling the payers and start the credentialing process.

Non-CAQH Applications

Some payers do not accept CAQH ProView and will send an application by mail, fax, or e-mail. Once the application is received, complete the application and return it to the payer with *copies* of the provider's documents. It is a good habit to make a copy of the application before sending it to have it on hand if the payer states he or she cannot find the application or if he or she needs a piece of the application, such as an attachment. Send the application using a means for tracking. (USPS, UPS, and FedEx all have tracking options available.) Insurance companies have no way to track your application until it is scanned into their system, which may take two or three weeks. Occasionally payers misplace applications; thus, tracking numbers come in handy to find the application and start the expediting process.

Following Up on Application Status

After submitting credentialing applications to payers by mail, fax, or e-mail, begin following up on the progress of your application every two weeks. Depending on the payer's workload, by two weeks the payer should have received and begun to review the application. When you start following up on the process of your payer's credentialing, you will want to make sure to take clear notes of all calls and e-mails between you and the payers. If anything comes up as missing, you will have notes of the operator you spoke with, when the application was sent, and the tracking number.

CMS and PECOS

The Centers for Medicare & Medicaid Services (CMS) created an Internet-based service, the Provider Enrollment, Chain, and Ownership System (PECOS), which can be used in lieu of a paper Medicare enrollment application (for example: 855I, 855R, 855B, etc.) to make updates to individual or group information. Begin by registering in the Identity and Access Management System (I&A) first, where you will obtain a username and password to log in to PECOS. You can follow up on the status of your application through PECOS. If you do decide to complete a paper application and submit to Medicare, call and verify with Medicare which administration company is handling the processing of the application.[1]

Access to PECOS is available at https://pecos.cms.hhs.gov/pecos/login.do#headingLv1.

Summary of Payer Credentialing

Before they are able to receive payment from government and private payers, healthcare providers must submit extensive data to prove that they have the proper credentials to render medical services to patients. The process is ongoing, because licensing and certifications have expirations and renewal requirements. The credentialer must gather and maintain the information. This section offers helpful pointers and forms for the process.

CONCLUSION

Credentialing is vital to functioning in the healthcare arena. It is the fundamental step in ensuring quality for the patient by verifying a doctor's qualifications. It allows patients confidently to place their trust in their chosen healthcare providers.

For the provider, credentialing is the primary method for receiving payment for their services. Physicians and other healthcare professionals must gain privileges to serve on a hospital's medical staff. Payers must have verification of the provider's qualifications to enter a contract for reimbursement for his or her services.

This chapter has provided the necessary information to achieve the tasks involved in ensuring a professional's credentials.

NOTES

1. Centers for Medicare and Medicaid Services. The Basics of Internet-Based Provider Enrollment, Chain, and Ownership System (PECOS) for Physicians and Non-Physician Practitioners. *Medicare Learning Network.* https://www.cms.gov/Outreach-and-Education/Medicare-Learning-Network-MLN/MLNProducts/downloads/MEDEnroll_PECOS_PhysNonPhys_FactSheet_ICN903764.pdf. Published December 2015. Accessed January 25, 2016.

CHAPTER 3

The Pros and Cons of Outsourcing Credentialing

The credentialing process is one of great import to private practices' and hospitals' employed physician networks (EPNs). Too often, credentialing is either performed haphazardly or is an afterthought to the signing of a physician's or advanced practice professional's (APP; i.e., nurse practitioner or physician assistant) contract. Truthfully, the two processes (the employment of a practitioner and credentialing) should synchronize so that the practitioner "participates" in most, if not all, of the system's payer contracts at the time that he or she begins seeing patients. Unfortunately, the coordination seldom happens.

Given the importance of credentialing physicians vis-à-vis reimbursement to the enterprise, it is a wonder that the credentialing process remains a stepchild in the operational function of the business. When providers see patients, and they are not credentialed, the enterprise runs the risk of either appealing denied claims (because the provider would be "out of network") or holding claims and submitting them once the provider is credentialed. For instance, with Medicare, providers can capture charges retrospectively for up to one (1) year before "timely filing" barriers are reached. This inefficiency builds unnecessary burden into the operations of the system's revenue cycle.

Credentialing is a detail-oriented endeavor requiring months to reach fruition, even when the process progresses smoothly. Healthcare entities should evaluate their credentialing process, procedures, and people to ensure that practitioners are added to insurance panels efficiently. Included in that evaluation should be the consideration of the positives and negatives of outsourcing credentialing.

The predicate to outsourcing, of course, requires that the company or person whom you engage in an outsourced model is fundamentally exceptional at credentialing and has an attention to detail that surpasses speed.

PROS: THE CASE FOR OUTSOURCING

Stop Gap

Outsourcing can be deployed effectively as a stop gap measure when there is a break in employment of credentialing staff (e.g., termination of a staff member, medical or other leave, etc.). Outsourcing as a stop gap provides a semblance of continuity to ensure that the process of enrolling physicians and APPs continues unabated. With quality "replacement" staff, healthcare enterprises can continue credentialing providers and expediting the protocol to confirm that there is no breach in the continuum.

The departure of a staff member, regardless of his or her skills in credentialing (e.g., strong vs. weak), without a suitable backup can present major challenges to onboarding and getting physicians paneled, which can ultimately negatively impact revenue.

Economies of Scale

Farming credentialing to a business/vendor that has the human capital bandwidth and structured processes and procedures to credential can be a reason to outsource. Companies that specialize, or have a service line with a specialty in credentialing, should bring to the table efficiency in process and structure because of their experience due to volume or their specialization in the multitude of steps that comprise the credentialing continuum.

Reduced Staffing Costs

The reduction of staffing costs may be a permanent or temporary solution. Outsourcing credentialing may make financial sense when the carrying cost of employees exceeds the cost to outsource. For instance, in the example below Hospital X has three employees who handle credentialing for its EPN. Table 3.1 identifies the employee costs of the in-house credentialing function.

TABLE 3.1: Hospital X—Current Employee Costs of the Credentialing Department

Hospital X Current Employee Costs of the Credentialing Department			
	Base Comp	**Benefits/ Taxes**	**Total EE Cost**
Suzy Q	$25,000	20%	$30,000
Janie Y	$27,500	20%	$33,000
Rupert M	$30,000	20%	$36,000
		Total:	$99,000

It costs Hospital X nearly $100,000 to manage the credentialing of the physicians and APPs in the enterprise. However, Schmoe Credentialing Corp has indicated that they could perform the credentialing for $75,000 per year, as Table 3.2 illustrates.

TABLE 3.2: External Credentialing Company Cost

Schmoe Credentialing Corp	
Cost:	$75,000

The obvious result is that Hospital X can save money by farming out their credentialing. According to Schmoe Credentialing, Hospital X can also gain efficiencies, accuracy, and speed (see Table 3.3).

TABLE 3.3: Hospital X—Savings by Outsourcing External Credentialing Services

Hospital X Current Employee Costs of the Credentialing Department			
	Base Comp	**Benefits/ Taxes**	**Total EE Cost**
Suzy Q	$25,000	20%	$30,000
Janie Y	$27,500	20%	$33,000
Rupert M	$30,000	20%	$36,000
		Total:	$99,000
Schmoe Credentialing Corp			
Cost:			$75,000
Savings:			$24,000

While Hospital X might save upwards of $24,000 per year by outsourcing, they may also elect to supplement (if necessary) their staff using Schmoe's Credentialing processes, or they may keep a lower-cost employee and contract much of the credentialing work to Schmoe Credentialing, thereby saving on overhead. As Figure 3.1 illustrates, when Hospital X's total employment costs pass $75,000, outsourcing becomes a more attractive financial option based on Schmoe's pricing.

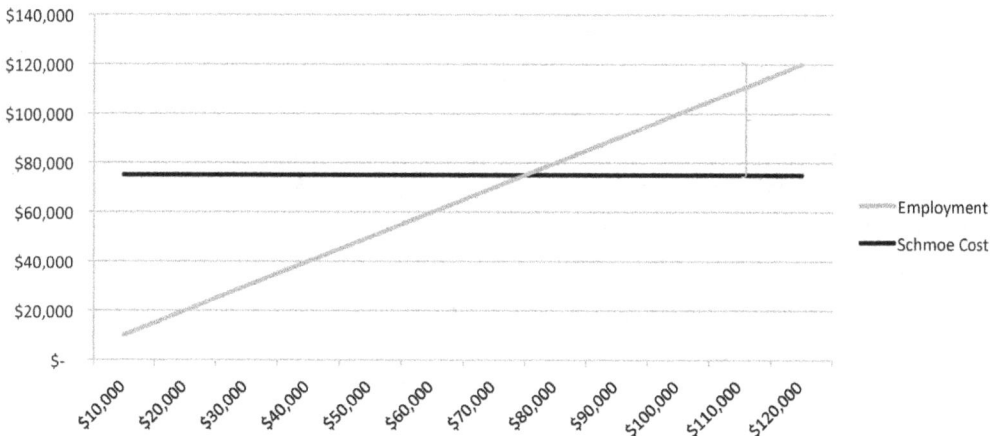

*Black line signifies Schmoe's cost to credential.
*Gray line equates to the practice or system's cost for employing credentialing staff.
*Intersection of gray and black lines designates the point where the cost to employ staff exceeds the cost to outsource.

FIGURE 3.1: Cost/Benefit of Outsourcing

Adjunct to Current Staff

As referenced above, outsourcing may be a viable and ongoing option adjunctive to current staffing. If there is an influx of providers who require credentialing, and insufficient staff to handle the workload, outsourcing to the right partner may help systems through the volume of new providers awaiting credentialing. When the immediate demand has waned, or the process is brought to the point where the paperwork is submitted to payers, and the waiting game ensues, the system might elect to scale back resources (and costs) to manage the remainder of the process in house.

Reduced Management Burden

Outsourcing should, theoretically, reduce managerial headaches and burdens. Outsourcing places the hiring/firing, raises, time off, and other management of staff burdens squarely on the outsourced vendor. For the enterprise, this relief purchases a level of freedom since they no longer have built-in and ever-increasing costs of carrying a staff member(s). However, outsourcing could negatively impact an enterprise if the contractor's staff is substandard, contentious, or not adequately screened or managed by the vendor.

CONS: THE CASE AGAINST OUTSOURCING

Expense Exceeds Staffing Costs

The cost of credentialing, both indirect and direct, should be measured with frequency (e.g., annually). Health systems that use third-party vendors for their credentialing may take an out-of-sight, out-of-mind approach to this important process. What can happen if the relationship is not managed carefully is that systems fail to see, as time passes, that they are paying more for credentialing services than they would pay if they had hired and managed their staff. That is, there could be cost creep as time passes in the relationship.

Although increases in cost may not occur frequently, there is the real prospect that systems that have outsourced the credentialing function may overlook its management of the costs, given the myriad more expensive programs that demand oversight.

The converse, though, might be that a health system is willing to pay a premium, however that is measured, to ensure continuity and the benefit of a sound credentialing program that is already in place and delivering solid results.

Also, it bears noting that transitioning credentialing to an outside firm, even if in a hybrid model, may create a lapse in the process unless there is a certain amount of overlap, with both the outsourcing firm and the employees working at the same time. But the transition may leave staff less willing to assist if they believe that their jobs and livelihoods are in jeopardy.

Loss of Control

Outsourcing the credentialing function removes a certain level of control from the health system. System executives are essentially divesting themselves of a very important cog in the provider onboarding and reimbursement processes by outsourcing. Outsourcing companies should provide updates as to credentialing status, constantly offering the health system's C-Suite input as to the status of providers in progress.

DUE DILIGENCE OF VENDORS

If a decision is posited to outsource or partner with a credentialing vendor, due diligence must be deployed in the vetting process to ensure that the new partner has a strong history of obtaining results and has rigorous processes and procedures in place that guarantee results. Due diligence requires background research, reference calls with current clients, review of fees in comparison to those of competitors, review of the partnership contract, and a candid discussion regarding any terminated relationships the vendor has had. Thorough vetting is essential because parsing out the credentialing process means effectively subcontracting a component in the revenue cycle process.

Vendor due diligence mandates discussion regarding background checks of vendor staff, tenure of the staff, specializing, reporting to the system, and process. It also requires, of course, that the partner company or person whom the enterprise engages is fundamentally exceptional at credentialing, demonstrating proven results.

If vetting is not thoroughly performed, and contracts are signed, health systems will not know until the vendor is engaged that the project was oversold, over promised, and under delivered. At that point, it may be too late.

Concerning the expense of staffing, there is the prospect that if no major errors occur when the vendor is engaged (or they are not reported), the relationship between the system and the vendor will continue with little oversight from the system. Again, the process may be considered by the health system to be "automatic," and so they abrogate the responsibility of managing and measuring the value and return of the credentialing vendor.

Complexity of Process

Credentialing, in theory, is straightforward. However, in practice it involves many variables and requires patience, diligence, and careful attention to detail. Without structure, the credentialing process can become an overwhelming behemoth of tasks, chores, and follow-up.

Partner vendors must have good, documented steps; checks and balances; timelines; and follow-up deployed. The checkpoints become more important in relation to the larger number of providers to be credentialed, because ostensibly the providers will be in different stages of credentialing.

If a vendor is engaged, there will be a large amount of data and files handed over to the vendor to use on behalf of the enterprise. Depending on how the credentialing staff of the enterprise manage the data and processes, this handoff can be cumbersome and problematic to the efficient credentialing of providers.

CONCLUSION

Suffice it to say, credentialing is an important and often undervalued component in a health system's onboarding of providers, and it is a baseline piece of the revenue cycle.

Whether credentialing for the hospital or employed model, the process historically has been the abused member of the family.

Systems should strengthen the credentialing process either through outsourcing or bolstering internal resources. Evaluation of the best approach, whether pure outsourcing, employing staff, or creating a hybrid approach, requires analysis and diligence by senior management. The end goal should be a solution that manages costs, strengthens core processes and procedures, and ensures continuity of the onboarding process.

While one methodology might appeal to a system, there are any number of approaches to conquering the problem of credentialing. Credentialing may not be a zero-sum proposition. Healthcare enterprises might opt for a hybrid approach to credentialing by supplementing current staff when inundated and flexing back down when the urgency and demand have subsided.

The key in whatever approach is deployed is to ensure accuracy and continuity of process and procedures. Whatever the case, enterprises should evaluate the pros and cons to outsourcing credentialing to ensure they are getting the most efficient and cost-effective process possible to confirm that providers are paneled with their payers.

CHAPTER 4

Regulatory Requirements

The Health Care Quality Improvement Act of 1986 was enacted to reduce medical errors and to protect the public. The purposes of the Act are outlined as follows:
1. to reduce the occurrence of medical malpractice;
2. to improve the quality of medical care;
3. to restrict the incompetent physicians to move from one state to another; and
4. to remedy the problems through effective professional peer review.[1]

HEALTH CARE QUALITY IMPROVEMENT ACT

The Health Care Quality Improvement Act of 1986 is, obstensibly, meant to protect the public from incompetent physicians by allowing those physicians on peer-review committees to communicate in an open and honest environment and thus weed out imcompetent physicians, without the specter of a retaliatory lawsuit by the reviewed physician.[2] The Act requires the reporting of certain adverse actions to the NPDB:
- a professional review action that adversely affects a physician's or dentist's clinical privileges for more than 30 days and is based upon the physician's or dentist's professional competence or professional conduct; and
- the voluntary surrender of clinical privileges by a physician or dentist who is under investigation relating to questions of professional competence or conduct, or in return for no investigation or professional review action being conducted.

PROFESSIONAL REVIEW ACTION

A professional review action includes denying, reducing, restricting, revoking, and suspending privileges, and it also includes a decision not to renew clinical privileges if the action is based on the physician's or dentist's professional competence or conduct.

Hospitals must submit adverse action reports to the appropriate state licensing board within 15 days of final board action in the case of an adverse action or within 15 days of the date the physician surrenders his or her clinical privileges. These reports must be submitted electronically to the NPDB as an adverse action report. Within 15 days, a printed copy of the electronic report must be forwarded to the state medical licensing board.

Revisions to previously reported adverse actions must also be reported. For example, if a physician's clinical privileges are reinstated after a 45-day suspension, both the suspension and the reinstatement must be reported.

ONGOING PROFESSIONAL EVALUATION

In 2008, TJC implemented a new standard requiring a detailed evaluation of practitioners' professional performance as a part of the credentialing and privileging process in a healthcare organization.

Ongoing Professional Practice Evaluation (OPPE) is intended as a means of evaluating professional performance on an ongoing basis as part of the effort to monitor professional competency, to identify opportunities for performance improvement by individual practitioners, and to use objective data in decisions regarding reappointment of practice privileges.

Once a provider has achieved practice privileges in a healthcare organization, TJC requires that performance data be collected, with evaluation of the provider conducted more frequently than annually. Evaluation done annually or less frequently is considered by TJC as "periodic," not "ongoing."

FOCUSED PROFESSIONAL EVALUATION

Focused Professional Practice Evaluation (FPPE) involves more specific and time-limited monitoring of a provider's practice performance when a provider is initially granted practice privileges, when new privileges are requested for an already privileged provider, and when performance shortfalls involving a privileged provider are identified (through the OPPE processor or by any other means such as complaints or significant departure from accepted practice).

TJC does not specify the length for a time period of FPPE. Therefore, each entity may choose the period of time for each FPPE episode; however, the FPPE process should have the following attributes:
1. be clearly defined and documented with specific criteria and a monitoring plan;
2. be of fixed duration; and
3. have predetermined measures or conditions for acceptable performance.

FPPE monitoring sessions for periods of three to six months are advised. For infrequently performed services, longer periods of monitoring, such as 12 months, may be warranted. An alternative approach for infrequently performed services may be the monitoring of a predetermined number of service events, rather than the monitoring of a prescribed period of time.

The duration and scope of FPPE monitoring may also be adjusted for the level of documented training and experience of a practitioner, with shorter monitoring periods or fewer service events for more experienced practitioners. All practitioners must be subjected to FPPE for new privileges, even those with extensive prior experience at other healthcare organizations.

All of the reporting and monitoring listed above assures the safety and quality of treatment rendered to patients nationwide.

CONCLUSION

This chapter has addressed the Health Care Quality Improvement Act, the professional review action, ongoing professional evaluation, and focused professional evaluation. The intent of these is to protect the public from being subject to malpractice and to improve patient care through a structured professional peer-to-peer review process.

NOTES

1. Healthcare Quality Improvement Act Law & Legal Definition. *USLegal.com*. http://definitions.uslegal.com/h/healthcare-quality-improvement-act/. Accessed January 11, 2016.
2. The Health Care Quality Improvement Act of 1986. *HCQIA*. http://www.hcqia.net/. Accessed January 11, 2016.

CHAPTER 5

Automated Payer and Medical Staff Credentialing Systems

In the past, credentialing procedures were largely dependent on manual processes that were tedious and overwhelming. Individuals tasked with the responsibility of keeping the information up-to-date relied on complex spreadsheets, calendars, lists, and cumbersome reminder systems. Now, in today's complicated data-intensive environment, manual procedures cannot support an ever-evolving credentialing process, especially for larger healthcare systems. Timely, efficient workflow is crucial to effective credentialing and privileging. Inefficiencies and unorganized procedures can be detrimental to maintaining ongoing revenue streams, and they can also make more difficult the management of the exposure to risk.

Therefore, credentialing software that expedites and streamlines credentialing procedures is a critical component of the process. The best systems support an organized workflow and online applications, and they provide scanning, electronic filing, and storage. This chapter offers some suggestions for evaluating and selecting products.

BENEFITS OF AUTOMATED CREDENTIALING SYSTEMS

There are a variety of systems that assist with compliance with regulatory requirements, including management of the FPPE and OPPE.

Workflow is optimized with system-generated employee work lists, expirables tracking, and automated verification, as well as integrated and seamless access to the NPDB. Online privilege forms enhance productivity by assisting with the management of delineation of privileges.

Automated credentialing review and processes increase the productivity of the credentialing staff members. In addition, timeliness and accuracy increase with an efficient automatic credentialing system. A good system also fosters prompt response times and appropriate decision making. Robust report capability to support quality initiatives for competency is another component of an efficient automatic credentialing system.

An effective credentialing system will enable staff to manage all facets of the credentialing process and to meet all regulatory requirements as indicated.

SELECTING AN AUTOMATED CREDENTIALING SYSTEM

The selection of the appropriate system for your organization begins with a request for proposals (RFP). RFPs should only be sent to vendors who have Web-based solutions. Automated application completion and document management systems also are critical features. The best systems will have automated reminders and alerts for expirables. Robust reporting to support privileging functions and regulatory requirements are additional essential features. The following are questions to include in your RFP:

1. Describe your organization.
2. Is the product software or a Web-based application? Explain.
3. How much does it cost? Explain.
4. How is it installed? Explain.
5. Does the product record, store, and report all data necessary to appoint, privilege, and credential healthcare providers? Explain.
6. Does the product work on every HMO, PPO, credentialing, and privileging application? Elaborate.
7. What technology platform is required for the solution?
8. Is your organization a CVO or outsourcing company?
9. How long does installing and training take?
10. Will my information stay confidential?

After the proposals have been narrowed down and all of the presentations are done, it is a good idea to request a client list from the vendor finalists. Then perform due diligence by contacting each of the clients to learn about their experiences with the system.

CONCLUSION

The right selection of an automated credentialing system will provide a solid foundation for credentialing and privileging that will be easy to manage, will monitor key performance indicators, and will maintain compliance with all regulatory requirements. But don't take the vendor's word for their system's functionality and reliability. Rather, ask existing clients what they think about the system and whether they would purchase the same solution again. The cost of the system will be offset by the increase in productivity and the reduction in the time that it takes to process medical staff appointments and reappointments.

CHAPTER 6

Training for the Credentialing Function

Having worked with EPN groups over the past several years, I have seen hundreds of thousands of dollars being adjusted off organizations' books because of inefficient credentialing policy and procedures. The lack of credentialing policy and procedures results in lost revenue at a time when hospitals need every dollar to thrive—and even, in some cases, survive!

STARTING STRONG

In many institutions, hospital administrators face a shortage of providers to meet their patient needs. Hiring involves searches that encompass interviews, reference checking, and negotiations. The arrangements can be for employment in the hospital or for acceptance as a member of the medical staff. However, once a provider has been hired, the offer is contingent on obtaining medical staff privileges, a process that can take weeks depending on the time required to obtain all of the information needed on the application.

As presented in Chapter 2, the next step after granting staff privileges is for the hospital to obtain Medicare, Railroad Medicare, Medicaid, and TriCare billing provider numbers under the hospital's Tax Identification Number (TID#). Many states require providers to have Medicare and Medicaid provider numbers before credentialing can began for Blue Cross Blue Shield, Aetna, Cigna, UnitedHealthcare, and others. The credentialing process can take 90 to 120 days to obtain an effective date for a provider to be able to treat patients. Providers who do not have an effective date with a payer will not be compensated for their services. Therefore, the charges generated will have to be written off for lack of obtaining the required credentialing. Many hospital administrators will allow providers to start seeing patients before completing the payer contracting and credentialing. This action results in the financial office having to write off booked revenue for the services. Hospital administration should become fully aware that the contracting and credentialing process must be complete before patient treatment begins, or the charges for treatment will not be reimbursed.

Hospital administration should have a policy in place that does not allow a provider to start working until all credentialing is completed and the effective dates are issued. Having this policy will provide an incentive for the provider to supply all the necessary information required for credentialing in a timely period. In cases of employed physicians, many are placed on the monthly payroll and are allowed to start seeing patients. However, the payers will not reimburse for their services until they are properly credentialed. The result of this discrepancy is a huge financial drain on the hospital's financial system, because salary dollars go out without the subsequent receivables to offset them.

One exception to the policy for completion of credentialing before practicing in the hospital is when there is a need for providers to see patients in a community and there are no other providers to perform them. When this occurs, the hospital should be aware they are providing free services.

STAFF PREPARATION AND TRAINING

Hospital administration should recognize the importance of hiring well-trained and experienced staff to handle provider credentialing. Too often, staff must find their way through the maze of information and self-train by trial and error. Training of credentialing personnel should encompass the following:

1. Hire an adequate number of support staff for the credentialing workload.
2. Educate the support staff on the credentialing requirements of government payers, commercial payers, and so on.
3. Provide adequate and appropriate tools (software or automated applications) for attaining and maintaining information.
4. Enable staff to attain credentialing certifications.[1]
5. Have the CFO conduct weekly meetings with credentialing staff to stay apprised of ongoing progress.

Hospital administrators must recognize the importance of having the credentialing department function at the highest level of knowledge to complete the credentialing correctly and timely. Often, staff members are assigned this responsibility without prior training. Allowing untrained staff to perform these duties will result in the rejection of credentialing applications and their return for incomplete information. Credentialing parties must understand the questions to fill in the blanks appropriately.

If payer credentialing is not given priority and staff given the resources and training to make sure the providers are credentialed and have effective dates to begin treating patients, hospitals will continue to forfeit much-needed revenue.

CHANGES IN MEDICARE

Reassignment of Medicare is another challenge for ongoing credentialing. Periodically, Medicare sends letters requesting the providers to update their reassignment information. Often the letter is sent to a provider's home or office address. In this event, the letter is not likely to get to the person performing the credentialing. If the reassignment information is not received by Medicare in a timely manner, the provider's services will not be paid. Many months can pass until someone checks on the provider's accounts receivable and learns that he or she is not being paid by Medicare. To reduce the likelihood of this occurring, the staff responsible for provider credentialing should update Medicare with the correct address of the department responsible for all information. This action will ensure that the reassignment letters are delivered to the appropriate staff for timely completion.

CONCLUSION

Training of staff members for the credentialing function starts at the top—in the office of the hospital administrator. The C-Suite and the medical staff should understand from the outset of the hiring function that privileges are contingent on the completion of credentialing, and the ability to receive payment for services is the foundation of the employment arrangement. The executive officers should know the importance of coordinating the timing of employment with the completion of the necessary stages of credentialing.

The financial office must stay on top of the status of the medical staff and be apprised of the credentialing progress. The responsibilities are ongoing, as renewals and updates continue throughout the calendar and over the years.

Training must be in place and advancement opportunities should be offered to staff members for the attainment of excellence and efficiency. The rewards of a knowledgeable and well-trained staff will be immeasurable, and the hospital will be strengthened financially by the support of the credentialing function.

NOTES

1. Note: The National Association Medical Staff Services (NAMSS) (see www.namss.org) offers guidance in becoming certified in credentialing. Some states have local and state organizations that offer education. There are two types of certification: Certified Provider Credentialing Specialist (CPCS) and Certified Professional Medical Services Management (CPMSM).

CHAPTER 7

Conclusion—The Importance of the Credentialing Process

The purpose of this book has been to provide the reader with complete and up-to-date information regarding the credentialing process. We conclude by expressing to those charged with this very important task the solemn responsibility that goes along with the many technical steps outlined herein.

PRIVILEGING

Quite simply, the privilege of serving others as a physician or another licensed healthcare provider is just that. It is an honor bestowed upon the very few who can demonstrate their capability and competency to take on this somber task as well as the burden of responsibility and accountability that go with it.

Hospitals and other credentialing bodies grant *privileges*, and that very term should be considered seriously by those involved in the credentialing of healthcare providers. The trust and confidence that come with being privileged to serve in this capacity are very fragile and can be easily disrupted if the credentialing process is not done correctly or thoroughly. Patients rely on credentialing professionals to keep them out of harm's way by making sure that those in whose hands they place both their physical and financial well-being are worthy of that trust.

Therefore, credentialing should always be done with the most important player in the healthcare system in mind: the patient. Medical science is a complex subject. While the Internet and other sources of information have served to make patients more informed consumers, it is difficult for most individuals to judge the validity of the information they receive from healthcare providers and to evaluate the abilities of those same providers to care for them in a high-quality, cost-efficient fashion. It is the credentialing professional's responsibility to serve patients in this way, and this responsibility should not be taken lightly.

TRANSPARENCY

The healthcare industry can use more transparency. This is true not only in the transparency of quality and price but also in the transparency of the credentialing process. Many practitioners have been protected by a credentialing system that loathes to share information with peers and with those most at risk from incompetent providers—namely, the patient population at large. While concerns over privacy and due process are legitimate, these concerns need not and should not take precedence over protecting the public from harm and exposing those who attempt to hide behind the far-too-often closed doors of the credentialing or decredentialing system.

REPORTING

National organizations such as the American Medical Association and their National Practitioner Database have gone a long way to circulate the names of incompetent providers while still protecting their identities and releasing them only to those with a need to know. That said, reporting to this database is often restricted by fears of legal retaliation on the part of the provider. Credentialing staff in provider or payer organizations need to resist this type of threat and always prioritize the safety of those who put their faith in the healthcare system.

CHANGES TO COME

Credentialing is a dynamic enterprise, and while many best practices and innovative solutions have been outlined in the preceding chapters, credentialing is a field that will surely benefit from more new ideas and better processes going forward. Keep your eye out for those novel concepts to come, and look for future editions of this book to provide updates and advances in the field.

SUMMARY

In summary, this book has outlined the differences between medical staff credentialing and payer credentialing. It has provided a detailed outline of best-practice processes for use in each credentialing type. It has covered the legal and regulatory requirements surrounding a high-performing credentialing program, and it has discussed ways that credentialing tasks can be automated or subjected to other technological or methodological innovations to improve quality and efficiency